FOURTH EDITION

stuttering and your child:

questions and answers

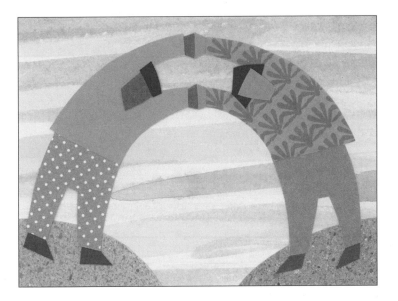

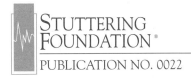

STUTTERING
FOUNDATION®

PUBLICATION NO. 0022

stuttering and your child:
questions and answers

Publication No. 0022

Third Edition—2002
Fourth Edition—2010

Published by

Stuttering Foundation of America
P. O. Box 11749
Memphis, Tennessee 38111-0749

Library of Congress Control Number: 2010932951
ISBN 978-0-933388-92-5

The Stuttering Foundation of America is a nonprofit
charitable organization dedicated to the prevention
and treatment of stuttering.

To Parents, Teachers, and All Those Concerned With Stuttering in the Young Child

This book represents up-to-date thoughts of seven leading authorities in the field of stuttering. All believe that early intervention is very important in the prevention of stuttering in the young child. Their names are listed below.

It was updated in 2010 to reflect the latest research on early childhood stuttering.

You will find answers to the questions most often asked by parents who are concerned about stuttering and their child. These answers will enable you to work with your child in ways that will contribute significantly to the healthy and normal development of fluency.

Jane Fraser
President

Stuttering Foundation of America

Edward G. Conture, Ph.D., Vanderbilt University
Richard F. Curlee, Ph.D., Professor Emeritus, University of Arizona
Hugo H. Gregory, Ph.D., Professor Emeritus, Northwestern University
Barry Guitar, Ph.D., University of Vermont
Lois A. Nelson, Ph.D., Professor Emeritus, University of Wisconsin
William H. Perkins, Ph.D., Professor Emeritus, University of Southern California
Dean E. Williams, Ph.D.,* University of Iowa

*Affiliation at the time chapter was written.

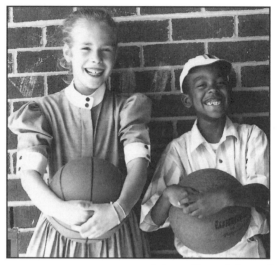

photo credit: paul diamond

contents

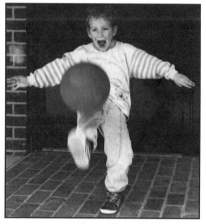

photo credit: paul diamond

Chapter 1

does my child stutter?

Richard F. Curlee, Ph.D.

He may. Many children begin to stutter during their pre-school years. This chapter answers some of the questions that parents often ask when they become concerned about their child's speech. As you read on and find out more about stuttering, you should be better able to answer this question.

What is "normal" speech?

"Normal" is what most of us hope we and our children are. "Normal" is what many of us think that we are seeing and hearing on TV. In fact,

"...what's normal always represents someone's judgment."

"normal" speech reflects a wide range of abilities. Some people speak barely above a whisper, others at a high volume. Some talk so rapidly that when we talk to them we can hardly get a word in edgewise. Still others hesitate and revise, repeat words and phrases "um" and "ah," and seem as if they are never going to finish their point. Most of us fall somewhere in between.

So, how can you tell if your child has crossed the line between "normal" and "abnormal"? First, it is important to remember that what's "normal" always represents someone's judgment. If you are concerned about your child's speech, that

1

means that you have made a judgment that he or she may not be "normal." This may be because your standards of "normal" are somewhat influenced by the superior speech that you observe from professional TV performers. As you read on and find out more about stuttering, you should be better able to decide if your expectations for your child's speech have been unrealistic or if you need to seek an evaluation of your child's speech from an expert in your area.

What is stuttering?

Stuttering involves the repetition, prolongation or blockage of a word or part of a word that a person is trying to say. Children who stutter know what they want to say. They may have said it hundreds, even thousands, of times before without stuttering. Yet, this time, in spite of all of their efforts, they are unable to say the word smoothly, effortlessly.

When children who stutter attempt to push through these disruptions of their speech, they may sometime blink their eyelids, turn their eyes to the side, turn their head to the side and, in other ways, struggle with speaking. Struggling to speak often does not begin until after a child has been stuttering for a while. Even though a child's use of physical tension and force to speak fluently is well-intentioned, it really makes it harder for them to speak and generally indicates that professional help is needed.

Does stuttering come and go?

In its initial stages, stuttering can be difficult to recognize because most children beginning to stutter often sound a lot like other children their age much of the time. At first, a child may only stutter occasionally. Stuttering occurs in some situations but not in others, often with no apparent rhyme or reason. Several days, perhaps a week or so, may go by with no problems. Then, without warning, a child may go through a period when he seems to stutter every time he opens his mouth.

Why does he stutter some times and not others?

Among young children especially, stuttering is very inconsistent. The amount and type of stuttering can vary from one day to another, from one situation to another. It can even vary during the same conversation. At present, no one knows why stuttering is so inconsistent.

We do know that stuttering often increases significantly when children are excited, excessively tired, apprehensive, feel rushed to talk or on display. Most of us, in fact, probably become more disfluent at such times. Occasionally, however, a young child will stutter severely, for no apparent reason, under the most calm, tranquil circumstances. The off and on nature of stuttering frustrates parents and has puzzled experts over the

"Stuttering rarely begins until after a child is speaking in short, meaningful sentences."

years. The frequency and severity of stuttering can change in unpredictable ways and is something to accept about the problem rather than becoming overly concerned about.

How can you recognize it?

There are several things you can look for in trying to determine if your child is beginning to stutter or is just fumbling around talking like many other children his age. First, children who stutter often have problems getting words started, and many of these disruptions occur at the beginning of sentences. When he stutters, he may also tend to repeat parts of words, for example, sounds or syllables, rather than whole words or phrases. In addition, they frequently repeat portions of words two or more times before they are able to say what they want. Sometimes a child may exaggerate or prolong a sound in a word. The child may seem to be stuck with no sound or word coming out, perhaps working hard at speaking, or look away just as his speech is disrupted. All of these are signs of stuttering; and if you observe your child talking this way, you should make an appointment for him to see someone in your area who specializes in helping those who stutter.

When does stuttering typically begin?

For most children, the risk for beginning to stutter increases from about their 2nd to 4th birthday, then decreases gradually until about the age of twelve. Often, stuttering begins gradually during the period when a child is acquiring language at a rapid rate. It rarely begins until after a child is speaking in short meaningful phrases, for example, "The boy is throwing the stick." In fact, most kids who stutter have been using sentences for some time, giving their parents no reason to suspect that they may not be developing speech normally before they begin to stutter.

Most people who are going to stutter will have begun before they reach their 5th birthday. Practically no one begins *after* age twelve. So, stuttering is really a developmental problem of early childhood.

How many people stutter?

There are more than 45 million people in the world today who stutter and approximately three million live in the United States.

Is stuttering a common problem?

It occurs often enough that most of us have had some experience with a neighbor, classmate, co-worker, or family member who stutters.

About 5% of all children are likely to stutter for several months or more at some time during their lives. Because stuttering runs in families, it is much more common in some families than others. For example, if a father or mother has ever stuttered, the chances that their children will stutter are three to five times greater than that for families in which neither parent has ever stuttered.

Which age group is most likely to stutter?

Stuttering is most prevalent among preschoolers, but decreases among older age groups. Nationwide, across all age groups, about ten persons in every thousand stutter. Among adults, about three in a thousand stutter severely and feel that their educational, vocational and social achievements have been affected by stuttering. In contrast, there are many prominent, successful people who have stuttered throughout most of their lives. Winston Churchill stuttered; so did Sir Isaac Newton, King George VI of England and writers Somerset Maugham and Budd Schulberg. So, too, do Bruce Willis, Carly Simon, Bob Love, James Earl Jones, and John Stossel.

Does stuttering look and sound the same in all children?

No more than any other two people look and sound alike. One dramatic way in which young children who stutter may differ is the way in which their speaking difficulties begin. As was noted earlier, stuttering typically begins gradually with periods of occasional stuttering mixed with periods of completely normal-sounding speech. For some children (perhaps as many as 30% of children who stutter) stuttering begins suddenly with obvious physical tensions and struggle, jaw tremors, frustration, even tears.

How does stuttering in children change with time?

"The off and on nature of stuttering frustrates parents and has puzzled experts over the years."

If stuttering persists, the nature of the child's speech disruptions often change. Some may begin to exhibit eye blinks, lip tremors, or head jerks during their speech disruptions. Often, such behavior disappears with time, gradually, just as it originally appeared. Other children may react to their speech disruptions with a great deal of frustration. These children are apt to avoid talking or even participating in situations where they think they might stutter. In time, their efforts to avoid stuttering are likely to become more of a problem than their disfluent speech ever could be. Without help, their anticipation and fear of stuttering can create a barrier which prevents them from doing what they are capable of doing.

Is stuttering something he's stuck with for life?

Probably not. Most children who begin to stutter gradually stop—perhaps as many as 80%. In fact, nearly half stop within six months of beginning to stutter. Of those children who continue to stutter as adults, about a third may stutter severely enough to adversely affect educational or vocational achievements. But even adults with chronic, severe stuttering problems can be helped to speak so that everyday communication need not be a significant problem.

My child has just begun to stutter, what should I do?

If your child has just begun to stutter, the odds are strongly in favor of his stopping. If he has been stuttering for some time, if he appears to struggle with his speech disfluencies, avoids talking in some situations or has expressed concern about his speech, you probably should seek professional assistance. Persistent, consistent stuttering is unlikely to disappear with age unless your child receives therapy for his problem.*

*See pages 62–64 for other factors that may also put your child at risk for stuttering.

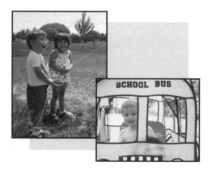

Things parents can do to help the child who stutters

Changes in Lifestyle

1) Accept your child. As much as possible, find ways to show your child that you love and value her and that you enjoy your time together.

2) Listen patiently. Listen to what your child says, not how it is said. Respond to the message rather than the stuttering.

Changes in Communication

1) Avoid filling in or speaking your child's thoughts and ideas. Let the words be his own.

2) Try neither to look away nor stare when your child talks. Keep natural eye contact while your child is talking.

3) Allow your child to complete what she is saying without interrupting.

4) Spend at least five minutes each day devoted to listening to and talking with your child in an unhurried, easy, relaxed manner.

5) After your child speaks, reply slowly and unhurriedly, using some of the same words.

   For example, if she says, "I s-s-see the b-b-b-bunny. He's cute." You reply in an easy relaxed way, "Oh yes, you see the bunny. He's cute."

6) Wait a second or so before responding to your child, for example: Child: "I like that doggie" (parent pauses about one second) Mother: "Yes, that is a nice doggie."

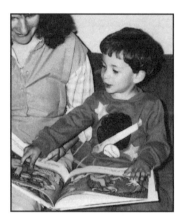

Chapter 2

why does my child stutter?

Edward G. Conture, Ph.D.

This is a question very frequently asked by parents: "Why does my child stutter?" No one knows for sure why children stutter. It makes perfect sense, however, that parents would want to know. It would seem that if "the cause" of stuttering could be identified, steps could be taken to eliminate it. The fact is that we do not need to answer that question in order to help your child.

What determines whether a child stutters?

While stuttering is often thought to have one cause, it may actually have several. Stuttering probably begins when a combination of factors comes together. For different young children, different things may lead to the same end: stuttering. Searching for one "cause" when several exist may become part of the problem rather than its solution.

There are many theories why children stutter, but none satisfactorily account for all that is known about stuttering. Children who stutter are no more apt to have psychological problems than children who don't stutter.

"Things that cause stuttering...are quite different from things that keep it going."

There is also no reason to believe that stuttering usually results from some emotional trauma or abnormal child rearing practice.

There is reason to believe, however, that for some children a predisposition to stutter may be transmitted genetically. It is also apparent that certain environmental conditions have to be present for stuttering to develop in some, if not all, children. The speech-language mechanism of these children appears to be vulnerable to disruptions in the flow of communication. The cause of such vulnerability is presently unknown, but some scientists now believe that some delays or differences in brain function may disrupt the rapid efficient planning and production of speech. Furthermore, there is also reason to believe that some children may react to such speech disruptions with apprehension and tension, making them worse, and increasing the likelihood that their stuttering will persist.

What causes stuttering? What keeps it going?

Things that cause stuttering may be, and probably are, quite different from things that keep it going, aggravate or make it worse. For example, if you mishandle a knife, you may cut your finger. The knife causes the cut and initial pain. Salt rubbed into the cut makes the pain continue or even worsen, but the salt does not cause the cut.

We still haven't found the "knife" that causes stuttering. However, we do know something about the "salt" that keeps it going, aggravates or makes it worse. Indeed, we will focus more on those things that keep stuttering going rather than those things that may have started or initially caused it. Why? Because, we *can change* those things that keep stuttering going.

Does stuttering begin after a sudden trauma?

"Parents are not to blame for stuttering..."

For most children who stutter, the onset of stuttering, as well as its recovery, appears to be gradual. Stuttering rarely if ever begins after a sudden trauma.

Occasionally, however, a child will have a very serious injury or unexpected experience just before. However, and this must be stressed, these types of sudden traumatic onsets of stuttering are *very few and far between*. In fact, most children who experience these sorts of sudden traumas or shocks DO NOT begin to stutter.

Who is to blame?

Parents are not to blame for stuttering. After years of study, we have found no reason to believe that the way parents rear their child causes stuttering.

On the other hand there are things that parents and the rest of the family can **do** that help the child's speech. For example,

- they can try to provide a calmer, less hurried lifestyle in the home.
- they can speak less hurriedly when talking to their child.
- they can allow their child to finish his thoughts.
- they can pause a second or so before responding to their child's questions;
- they can try not to talk for their child, and so forth.

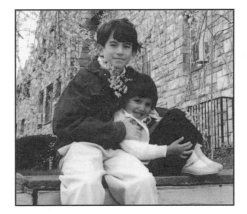

Do adults or parents sometimes hinder a child's speech?

On occasion, parents, brothers, sisters, aunts and uncles and the rest of the family can do things that **hinder** the child's speech; for example, finishing the child's sentences, interrupting the child while he is talking, encouraging or requiring him to talk rapidly, speaking to the child using a rapid rate of speech, and maintaining an overly rapid lifestyle within the home.

None of the things a listener or parent does that may hinder a child's fluent speech make that individual a bad person or parent. However, these types of behavior make it difficult for a child who is already having trouble establishing his speech fluency. If parents change some things in the home (for example, slowing down their rate of speech when the child stutters, decreasing the number of times they ask the child to perform for or give little plays or speeches to people visiting the home), they can do a lot to help.

What part do the child's abilities play?

Each child has his or her strengths and weaknesses. Within one family, each child may be very different. And, after all, wouldn't it be a boring world if we were all the same? Parents need to realize that each of their children has unique abilities and that some of these may be influenced very little by things you as parents may do (even though, as we said above, there are some things that you do that can help or hinder the child's development of fluent speech).

Do problems with the brain cause stuttering?

Recent publications of brain imaging activity and structure suggest that there may be subtle differences in the brain activity and/or structure in some adults who stutter. It is fair to say, though, that more research in this area is needed. More people and areas of brain activity will need to be studied before reaching firmer conclusions. We do know that the brain has some sort of involvement with stuttered speech because it is involved with non-stuttered speech! What we still do not know, however, is how any differences in brain activity in people who stutter may influence or cause the actual stuttered speech behavior we see and hear.

Things That HELP

Lifestyle

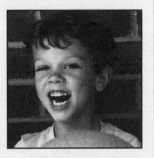

1) Provide a calm, unhurried lifestyle in the home as much as possible.
2) Turn off the television, radio, stereo and computer during dinnertime. This is a time for family conversation, not listening to television or radio programs or playing video/computer games.
3) When the child gets in the car after school, minimize questioning of him or her, let your child begin the talking and let him talk about what is on his mind.
4) When your child talks, try not to talk for the child or rush her to finish her thoughts.

Communication

1) Speak less hurriedly when talking to the child, particularly when they are stuttering a lot.
2) Allow the child to finish his thoughts.
3) Pause a second or so before responding to the child's questions or comments.
4) If your child begins to talk to you while you are doing things that require concentration (for example, driving a car, using a knife to cut vegetables), tell him that you can't look away right now but that you are listening to him and that he has your attention.

Things that HINDER

Lifestyle

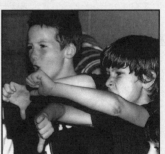

1) Maintaining an overly rapid lifestyle within the home (or constantly feeling or acting as if "everything had to be done yesterday").
2) Making her give little speeches, plays or read aloud to visiting friends, relatives or neighbors.

Communication

1) Finishing the child's sentences.
2) Rushing the child to finish his thoughts or sentences.
3) Interrupting the child while she is talking.
4) Encouraging or requiring him to talk rapidly, precisely and maturely at all times.
5) Frequently correcting, criticizing, or trying to change the way she talks or pronounces sounds or words, or telling the child to "talk normal."
6) Speaking to the child using a rapid rate of speech, especially while telling him to slow down his own rate of speaking!

If my child "imitates" someone else's stuttering, will he become a stutterer?

We've never heard of anyone who began to stutter through living with and imitating a stutterer! Further, normally fluent speech clinicians who have worked with literally hundreds of individuals who stutter—through all their exposure to stuttering—have not "picked-up" nor developed the problem. Most stutterers began stuttering without ever having heard anyone else stutter.

The imitation myth dies hard. In part, the myth's refusal to die relates to our belief that children copy the habits of their elders like so many little copy machines. While this copying may be at least partially true for certain behaviors, it is not true for stuttering.

Why do some children begin to stutter after a fairly normal period of speech and language development?

Some children who stutter struggle with their speech and language right from the beginning while others seemingly have little trouble with speech until they start to stutter. Most, however, only start stuttering after they have begun to use sentences to express their ideas (sometime after 2 years of age).

No one knows for sure why some children begin to stutter after a period of seemingly normal speech development. One idea is that the various abilities a child needs for speaking develop at different rates. For example, it is not uncommon to find a child whose expressive or spoken language skills are superior but whose ability to speak with clarity, speed and precision is quite delayed. Perhaps this sort of developmental "mismatch" contributes to difficulties some children have maintaining smooth, easy speech after they have been talking normally for a while.

Why do more boys stutter than girls?

About three times as many boys as girls stutter. However, boys are more apt than girls to have other speech and language problems, too. This apparent difference in susceptibility to stuttering has been attributed to differences in boys' and girls' biological constitutions, physical maturation, and/or speech and language development, as well as to differences in parents' attitudes and expectations towards boys versus girls. The evidence is not sufficient for us to rule out any of these possible explanations with confidence.

Do children stutter on purpose?

In our experience this only happens when one child is ridiculing or mocking another child by

"...we know of no documented evidence to support claims that a youngster stutters on purpose."

overtly imitating the other child's stutterings. It is not fun to stutter, and few children appear interested or willing to do so if they have any choice in the matter.

It is possible, however, to think of two exceptions to the rule: (1) a child seeking parental attention (this is based on the premise that any attention is better than no attention at all); and (2) a child verbally "acting out" against the parents for some reason. But these possibilities are *quite rare*. Simply put, we know of no documented evidence to support claims that youngsters stutter on purpose. Instead, our clinical experience working with many, many of these children and their families is that if children who stutter could or would do anything on purpose, it would be to speak more fluently.

Can stuttering be caused by moving?

It's been said that you can go 3000 miles and still remain where you are. Indeed the heaviest baggage you take with you when you travel is yourself. You may be moving to new surroundings but your old self and problems still follow you. The same goes for your child.

First, every year many families move across town, across or out of state without having their children begin or develop stuttering. Second, if moving were such a powerful influence on stuttering, we'd see much more stuttering, which we don't, in the children of families who work in the military. Third, we must once again distinguish between what *causes* and what *worsens* it. For example, let's assume the child's speech was already slow in its development and the child, for whatever reason, began to get concerned about meeting and making new friends, leaving old ones, and the like. If this were the case, the stage might be set for conditions that would disrupt fluent speech. The chances for disruptions increase even more if the child is tired because of the packing, the trip to the new house, and unpacking. Further, if the parents themselves—who are just as tired as their children or even more so—react to the move by becoming fatigued, overly stressed and unpleasant to be around, then the child may find it hard or unpleasant to talk with them. In this way, the move may *aggravate* an already existing or emerging problem. But by itself, moving does not cause stuttering.

Can starting school cause stuttering?

Beginning school is a time of excitement, a time of new challenges for all children. The young child must meet and deal with new friends and adults and learn to work and play in new surroundings. It is a time of uncertainty for all children as new relationships are being made, new skills tried out, and new rules being learned. While these events may make it hard for the young child to keep all his previous advances in speech development, they don't cause stuttering.

Should my child go to school with other children?

The excitement, the uncertainty and the stresses to perform that occur during the new school year may **aggravate** an existing or developing problem like salt rubbed into a wound. It is very important to realize, however, that your child's future lies with friends as much as with his elders. School is, therefore, an excellent place for him to learn how to deal with people his age. You can be of tremendous help to your child by supporting him as he learns how to play and work with other children at school.

"Children can't be reared in cocoons... like delicate houseplants; they have to be allowed to get excited, nervous or tired as the situation dictates.

16

Can too much excitement cause stuttering?

It's been said that too much of a good thing is no good. Excitement, which we all feel at various times, can be wonderfully stimulating; but for a young child, too much excitement for too long can be too much. While excited, the child may continuously run around inside and outside the house until dropping with fatigue, all the while jabbering at a 100 miles an hour. Very few parents could remain fluent if they acted like this!

No, excitement doesn't cause stuttering, but it can make it difficult for the young child to continue to speak fluently, particularly when he is talking fast while tired and competing with other talkers. We don't want our children to vegetate in the corner like a mushroom, nor do we want them to continually speed around like a bullet. Parents can and should help their child bring the excitement level down by quietly playing with him, speaking slowly themselves using a quiet tone of voice. If you try to be reasonably relaxed and not do things or speak in a hurry yourself, it will help your child to do the same.

Does my child stutter because of nervousness?

There is no evidence to prove that children who stutter are more nervous more often than usual, nor is there evidence to suggest that nervousness is the main or sole reason why children stutter, though it may aggravate the problem. Of course, if your child or any child is routinely reminded, told or **required** to speak maturely, precisely and quickly, he may feel under stress. Children can't be reared in cocoons or like delicate houseplants; they have to be allowed to get excited, nervous or tired as the situation dictates. These children, like all children, will experience situations in which they will get more nervous than usual. You can look for ways to help your child deal with these situations constructively and successfully.

A parting shot

We encourage you to routinely ask or focus on what you can do in the present and future rather than concentrating on what may have happened in the past. If you do this more often, you will be of tremendous help to your child.

17

how does our home life influence his stuttering?

Lois A. Nelson, Ph.D.

Should we treat him like our other children?

Yes, of course—with some exceptions. Just like you do, your child should think of himself as a "regular kid," a regular kid who just happens to stutter. To do this, he needs to be taught the standards of behavior, the social values, and the kinds of responsibility that you expect of your other children. Children are not helped to feel "regular" if they receive special treatment—whether the special treatment is because they stutter or for any other reason. Just because the child may stutter, he or she should not be allowed to avoid routine responsibilities. For example, this might involve emptying the trash, feeding the cat, straightening his room, and so forth as well as routine social behaviors, for example, saying hello to store attendants when with their parents.

Of course, you probably know that your own children differ from each other in many ways. Many parents comment that they discipline each child a little differently. They may problem-

"Sometimes parents expect too much from their child."

solve with one child but insist on a strict follow-the-rules system with another. They have discovered through experience that strategies which work with one child may be less effective with another.

What are some exceptions?

We know that the child who stutters may take more time to talk, and we hope you will try to be patient and listen until he finishes. You should try to ensure that the child has opportunities to express his ideas. Nevertheless, a child who stutters can and should learn to take turns talking and develop other social skills as well. Stuttering should not become an excuse for him to monopolize the conversation or interrupt the person who is talking. Again—and we can't stress this enough—the child who stutters should be given as much as possible, **all** the academic, learning, social, etc. experiences that any other child his or her age experiences.

Do we expect too much from our child?

Sometimes parents expect too much from their child. Children can feel pressured if they try, yet frequently fail, to meet mother's, father's or the family's expectations. Likewise, a child feels pressured if he does not live up to his own expectations. This kind of stress can aggravate stuttering.

Should we leave him with a babysitter?

Some children have a more difficult time than others when separated from their parents for an afternoon or evening. As much as possible, this decision should be made separately from the fact that your child stutters. Would you leave him with a sitter if he didn't stutter? If the answer is "yes," then feel free to leave him with the sitter.

As for any child, you will probably instruct the sitter about house rules, bedtime routines, and leave a telephone number where you can be

"Ask the sitter to be patient and listen to what your child says, not how he says it."

reached. Similarly, you can prepare the sitter on how to handle the situation if your child stutters. Calmly inform her ahead of time that your child may stutter, and briefly describe how his stuttering sounds and what it may look like. Use descriptive terms such as "he repeats the first syllable of a word" or "he has trouble getting the word started." Explain whatever it is the child actually does most of the time.

Since children often feel uncomfortable when they know they are being discussed, try to do this when the child is not present. If he happens to overhear you talking about his stuttering, he may feel that something is amiss. At that point, it would be wise to talk with him about it openly.

End your conversation with the babysitter by telling her what you say and do when your child stutters. For example, you might say, "we wait for him to say the word himself and try not to finish words or sentences for him; we try not to cut him off or get him to talk less; we don't imitate his stuttering or tease him; and we look at him as he talks." You could explain the situations in which he is likely to stutter more, such as when he gets really excited, overly tired, is hurried, describes objects and events outside the house, or is asked many questions. Ask the sitter to be patient and listen to what he says, not how he says it.

What Babysitters Can Do to Help

Childcare/rearing
1) Treat the child who stutters like all the other children you babysit.
2) Don't let him get away with things that his brothers and sisters aren't allowed to do.

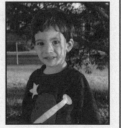

Communication
1) Be as patient as possible and pay attention to what the child says, not how he says it. Respond to the child's message.
2) Here are a few "don'ts" that will help:
   a) Don't finish words or sentences for him.
   b) Don't interrupt.
   c) Don't correct the way he talks, pronunciations, childhood grammar or any other mistakes in his speech.
   d) Don't keep the child from talking.

Does he need more rest than other children?

He may. Most of us make more mistakes when typing on our computer keyboard or in pronouncing words and expressing ideas clearly when we are tired, distressed or distracted. If fatigue appears to influence your child's speech, you may want to make doubly sure that he gets sufficient rest, and goes to bed and wakes up at reasonably consistent times.

Should my child have regular bedtime hours?

Consistency in bedtime helps any child adjust to a sleep schedule. Consistency also has value from another perspective. Children benefit from the order of daily routine: waking, dressing, mealtimes, and going to bed. They learn what to expect in their lives and when to expect it. This kind of structure reduces uncertainty in their lives. One caution: parents shouldn't be expected to follow an overly rigid schedule. Use your best judgment in making these decisions. While consistency is important, be flexible in your approach because daily circumstances change, requiring parents to adjust their schedule and that of their child. In other words, it is good to be consistent, but be flexible in doing so!

Does your family's lifestyle need to be changed?

Many parents find that their young child's stuttering increases when the family's lifestyle is fast-paced. Children differ considerably in their energy levels and the effect that a hurried family lifestyle has on them. Be guided by the unique nature of your child, and if slowing down the family's pace seems to help your child, then it is important for you to do.

Does my child who stutters need more attention?

Whether your child continually seeks, wants or needs additional attention depends partly on his feelings of self-worth, his personality/temperament, and his ability to entertain himself. Children value individual time with a parent. If your child stutters often, extra attention and listening time are likely to help him feel better about the talking he does and about his importance to you.

Providing a child opportunity for uninterrupted listening time can markedly decrease stuttering in very young children. When a child expects to be and is interrupted by brothers and sisters, it is difficult for him to talk fluently. He feels pressured to talk quickly when he has to continually compete for Mom and Dad's attention.

Do I let him watch overly-exciting TV shows?

If a television show...appears too exciting for the child who stutters, it's probably too exciting for his brothers and sisters."

We hope not, particularly if he is a preschooler, especially just before bedtime. Many young children are easily excited by what they see and hear, and some shows actually frighten them. High excitement levels, from any source, may aggravate stuttering in children. Long after a child's speech has improved, he is still likely to stutter occasionally when he is under stress or highly excited. Parents tell us, "He is really talking well now. The only time he still stutters is when he gets excited." If a television show or any other experience appear too exciting for him, then it is too exciting for any of your other children as well.

Should we watch what he eats?

Children need a balanced diet in order to grow and be healthy. Your child's physician, public health nurses and hospital dieticians are excellent sources of information about adequate nutrition. Follow their advice and your own good judgment. Again, as with sleep, routine times, reasonably maintained, for breakfast, lunch and dinner also help provide children with consistency in their daily life and knowing what to expect and when.

What if my child is frequently inattentive, impulsive and/or hyperactive?

Some children exhibit behavior that parents and teachers describe as chronically active, restless, impulsive, impatient or distractible—to name only a few traits. These parents express concern that their child is truly inattentive as well as hyperactive. They also express the fear that this may hinder him both academically and socially. They find that their child's behavior frequently disrupts their home life and report that their efforts to cope with him are only partially effective. A few children who exhibit the above traits also stutter, and the parents worry that the hyperactivity contributes to the stuttering and vice versa.

If you are concerned about your child's apparently frequent inattentiveness, impulsiveness, hyperactivity (and related behaviors), you

"...some parents keep their house so tidy and clean they act like they are performing surgery rather than raising children in their home."

should contact your family physician or pediatrician and request that your child be evaluated by specialists in the area of Attention Deficit Disorder (ADD). If this diagnosis is made, then medical and/or psychological management precedes or at least should take place simultaneously with therapy for speech and language problems. Many states have a support group for parents or children with attention deficit hyperactive disorders (ADHD).

How neat should his room be?

It's not as much neatness as it is how the parent achieves it that is important here. It's how your child feels about keeping his room neat. How does your child respond to the reminders to pick up his things? Does he feel that you are nagging him? Does he feel overly pressured to comply? Most parents comment that they wonder if he's ever going to learn to be neat. Most children react to those reminders or comments with no observable effect on their speech or other behavior. Listen to what he says and how fluently he says it. Does he stutter more frequently or more severely whenever the appearance of his room is discussed? You may be more willing to re-evaluate your priorities about neatness if you discover that continually nagging him about neatness contributes to stuttering.

What if he is overly concerned with neatness and cleanliness?

Tidiness, cleanliness, and the like are fine, as long as they are not taken to extreme, by either the child or the child's parents. Some children are so concerned and worried about getting themselves or their clothes dirty, wrinkled, etc. that they routinely refuse or are reluctant to participate in daily life events, for example, going outside and playing with other children in their own yard. Likewise, such children may routinely want to rush home from daily activities, for example, playing in a park with his parents, because he has just gotten his hands or shirt a little bit soiled or wrinkled.

Some adjustments with the child and the child's home life may be considered when the child's desires to be orderly, tidy and clean becomes the focus of his and his parents' day. This is especially true when these behaviors get in the way of his and the family participating and enjoying routine activities like playing outside, playing with friends, and the like. It is not unusual to find that a child's persistent, strong concerns with tidiness and cleanliness are encouraged, demanded or modeled by one or both parents. It is as if some parents think they are performing surgery rather than raising children in their house!

Again, with neatness and cleanliness, it is helpful to strive for the middle ground, being neither too sloppy or dirty nor too clean or orderly. Talking about these issues with a health care professional, for example, your pediatrician or a child psychologist may also be of assistance. Achieving a balance, for your child, and yourself, in terms of orderliness and cleanliness is important, healthy and more relaxing than continually approaching your living space as a surgical suite!

What about fighting with other children?

Fighting seems to be part of learning to live with brothers and sisters and the neighborhood kids. Much as parents dislike it, children do and say mean things to each other. It's a reality. Children who stutter are just as likely to do and say mean things as other children. Some fighting among children is to be expected, and parents should not be overly concerned about this. In fact, continually acting as referee between your children's arguments should probably be lessened; let them sometimes settle their differences. This helps them develop normal, healthy independence from their parents.

What about fights and arguments between his mother and father?

Arguments between parents occur even in families where the father and mother have a very good relationship. Professionals such as psychologists and family counselors consider it important for children to discover that disagreements do not signal a loss of love or an impending divorce. They want the children to learn that arguing with someone doesn't diminish that person's caring for them.

But when verbal fighting between adults is nearly daily, chronic or becomes excessive or abusive, children can become alarmed. They feel vulnerable in these situations, and they are. Older children may be forced into the role of protector for one parent or peacemaker for the family. This kind of environment does not nurture the child's development. If fights and arguments in your family affect your child's stuttering, and you have been unsuccessful in coping with this problem, seek help from professionals, such as family counseling agencies.

His mother and father are thinking about separating. Will this aggravate his stuttering?

Perhaps, but it all depends on how the parents and child react. It may also affect many other things, such as his performance at school, playing with friends and so forth. But, if the relationship between his parents is already generating friction within the family, it may already have aggravated his stuttering.

It is the real or possible **change** in family life the child is reacting to as much as anything. What seems to be important is how the child reacts to the current family problem and what he expects to happen to him if his parents do separate. Do what you can to maintain stability in his life as well as your own.

**His mother and father are separated or divorced.
Will this hurt his stuttering?**

Separation and divorce in American families is not unusual. Although you may be especially concerned about your child who stutters, the emotional impact of the events leading to that decision will have influenced the entire family. Reassure your children, as much as possible, that they are loved, that they didn't cause the break, and that both parents will always remain their parents. Keep in mind that usually no single event in a child's life is responsible for maintaining stuttering.

I am a single parent. Does this influence his stuttering?

One main difference is that a single parent simply has no one with whom to share the stresses of daily living. Many single parents do a very good job of coping with these demands and this has a very good impact on the child. The ways in which a parent deals effectively with stress are likely to be ones the child learns to use in handling his own, whether there is one parent or both parents present.

Should anyone in the family correct his stuttering?

No. That doesn't really help. Even if the family member has the best intentions, the child who stutters seldom reacts to correcting as kind and helpful. He may get the message that he is not acceptable unless he speaks well. After all, if he were okay, why would everyone be trying to change the way he talks? Remember: if simply correcting his speech had worked, you probably wouldn't be reading this book now!

Should we let his younger or older brother and sister imitate his stuttering?

No. Imitation is a form of teasing. Teasing can hurt anyone especially when it's about behavior they cannot help doing. When teasing occurs, you can tell your children that imitating their brother's stuttering actually makes it harder for him to talk and might even make his stuttering worse. But do not scold them for teasing.

Instead, try to realize that you cannot stop teasing entirely and that you should not get overly concerned about it. After all, most of us were teased as children, at some point, and by and large, it had little lasting influence on us.

Should we have the TV, radio or stereo on during meal times?

"Meal times are family times, times to listen to...our children."

Definitely not. Children generally find it more difficult to talk when there is a lot of activity going on or when the computer, radio, TV or CD is being used in the same room. Background noise, music or speech forces the child into a form of competition and can contribute to breakdowns in his speech.

Meal times can be quite hectic with brothers and sisters verbally competing for Mom and Dad's attention. Children are bursting with things to tell and want to be heard. Parents find their attention divided between listening to their children and eating their food! If parents' attention is further divided by TV or radio programs, a child will quickly sense that his parents' interest is focused elsewhere and that one or both parents are only half-heartedly listening to him.

Turn off the radio, TV and stereo **during** meals, and family conversations; this will improve the situation. By not listening to or watching various media, talking during meal times should become less stressful and competitive for everyone—particularly those who may stutter. Mealtimes should be one of the best times for sharing the day's experiences and having an exchange of ideas.

If you must catch up on local, state, national or world news, do so before or after eating! Meal times are family times, times to listen, talk with and attend to our children!

what do I tell people about my child's stuttering?

Dean E. Williams, Ph.D.

How can I talk to my child about talking?

It helps when discussing stuttering with a child to explain it by using analogies taken from common experiences in his every day life. This approach enables the child to view stuttering not as something mysterious and scary but as something understandable and solvable. It also provides a common platform from which you and your child can understand what each is talking about. Such mutual understanding helps to get the child on a positive course for coping with his speech problem.

"Learning to talk is a big job for a little person."

Your child is learning new things every day. We know, but sometimes forget, that making mistakes is an essential part of learning. He can be helped to understand that he made mistakes when he learned to dress himself, when he learned to eat with a spoon, when he learned his A B C's, or to count, etc. But the mistakes were okay. They were a normal part of learning.

How can I reassure my child it's okay to make mistakes?

Learning to talk is a big job for a little person. It's very important with young children to view the stuttering as "making mistakes." He is repeating sounds and words. That's all right. Everyone makes mistakes as they learn to talk. Some make more than others—just as some children make more mistakes than others as they learn to count, or, to read, or to catch a ball, and so forth. (Examples used should correspond to your child's own interests.) Your child is probably making more mistakes than many children when he talks, but probably not as many as some of his friends as he learns other things. It helps to have this pointed out to him. His speech will undoubtedly develop all right. In the meantime, it's helpful to reassure your child that it's okay to make mistakes—that it is much more important to you that he talks and has fun talking. If he does this, then it will be easy for you to learn the things he thinks about, the way he feels, and the things he likes and doesn't like. Assure him that these are the important things about talking—not whether he makes mistakes as he learns how to talk.

What if my child is tensing and struggling as well as repeating sounds?

If your child is not only repeating sounds but also is tensing and struggling, you can follow the same kind of explanation as outlined above. However, there will be a need to add to the examples.

Let us say as an illustration that a child is learning to catch a ball. He's dropping the ball quite a bit. He doesn't like doing this, so he begins to tense up and "pounce" at the

> *"Some children focus on 'mistaking' rather than talking."*

ball. He begins to drop it more often. He is now trying hard "not to drop it." The same thing occurs when one begins to learn to ride a bicycle. Often the child will tense up to try "not to fall off." He will fall off more often. In a sense these children are "fighting the making of mistakes."

29

The same thing can happen if a child begins to believe he should not make mistakes while talking. In an effort to "not" make them, he physically tenses and struggles. This only makes talking more difficult. He can be helped to see that it is more beneficial to "go ahead and talk and stutter easily." This makes it easier for him to say what he wants to say.

What do I tell his brothers and his sisters about stuttering and about what they can do to help?

You can explain stuttering to his brothers and sisters in much the same way as you explain it to your child. He can be present or not when you explain it to them. There is nothing secretive about making mistakes and even fighting them— we all can give examples—even his brothers and sisters. Explained in this way, it makes it easier for

"Explain...in a matter-of-fact way...that he is stuttering some during this phase of learning to talk."

them to understand what they can do to be helpful. After all, if they were having difficulty learning an activity, they would want others: (1) to give them time to work through their mistakes; (2) to wait calmly and not interrupt them; and (3) not to jump in and do it for them. The same is true for a child who is stuttering (reacting to disruptions in his speech).

As a way to help, set up talking rules in your home. The talking rules apply to your child who stutters as well as to his brothers and sisters.

1) We don't interrupt each other as we are talking.
2) We take turns talking.
3) We don't talk for each other. Each does his own talking.

How should teasing be handled?

In addition to talking rules, I suggest that you establish a position about teasing. If discussions have been open about your child's stuttering problem, there should be a minimum of teasing. However, if teasing occurs by a brother or sister, it is easy to point out to them that if they worked hard on a math paper, for example, and then made many mistakes, they feel bad. They would then feel even worse if anyone teased them at that time. The same is true when they tease anyone else. You can set up a rule that in your family, one doesn't tease another about the way he or she does things. To do so only makes one feel sad. Teasing doesn't help one learn—and we are a family, and we are all trying to help each other.

What do I say to his friends?

Essentially, you can talk to them the same way I suggested you talk to his brothers and sisters. It is not unusual for a friend of your child to turn to you and ask "How come he talks that way?" or, "Why does he stutter?" Again, it is important when you answer your child's friend in an open, matter-of-fact way. Your child will likely be present. Your answer to the friend should be similar to the explanation that you gave to your child and to his brothers and sisters. Presenting similar explanations about stuttering to your child's friends enables you to handle any teasing by friends in the same way explained previously for brothers and sisters.

What do I say to the babysitter and to the people at the day care center?

Explain to adults who take care of your child, in a matter-of-fact way, that he is stuttering some during this phase of learning to talk. Make it clear to them that you want him to talk to them and you want them to talk to him. If you can help them view the stuttering as the making of mistakes, then it will be easier for them to see that he should be encouraged to express ideas just as any other child.

You also can help them understand that when disruptions occur, the child should be given the time he or she needs to work through them. Listeners should try not to hurry him or finish words or ideas for him. At the same time, he should receive the same discipline practices as any other child. Also, he can be helped to learn the same talking manners as any other child. He should learn to "take turns" in talking, and he should not interrupt, talk for, or finish words for anyone else— any more than they for him.

What Day Care Centers can do to help

General Practice

1) Treat the child who stutters the same as the other children at the center.
2) Don't let the child who stutters get away with things just because she stutters.
3) View the child's stuttering as having some disruptions in the normal learning process. This child should be encouraged to express ideas just as any other child at the center.
4) The child who stutters should receive the same disciple as any other child.

Communication

1) When he has disruptions in speech, allow him time to work through them;
   a) without listeners hurrying him;
   b) without listeners finishing words or ideas for him.
2) The child who stutters should learn the same talking manners as any other child; for example,
   a) taking turns talking;
   b) listening while others talk, and
   c) not interrupting others or finishing their words or ideas for them.

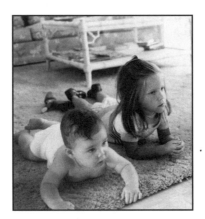

When his grandparents or his aunts and uncles ask, what should I say about his stuttering?

Try to adopt the same basic philosophy with close relatives we discussed above under ways to talk to your own child and to his brothers and sisters about stuttering. This enables all close family members to see the problem in the same way. It provides a common-sense approach that is readily understandable by all. This approach encourages all "family" to be consistent in the ways they react to the act of stuttering and to the child who is doing it.

What should I do if my child stutters in public and if a stranger comments about it?

At times this may be difficult, but remember when a child stutters, he is talking—and when he is talking, he is trying—although clumsily at times—to send you a message. Therefore, attend to, and work to interpret the child's message. Don't get sidetracked by the static, the hesitations, that may be accompanying the child's message.

If he stutters in public, or anywhere else for that matter, pay attention to and respond to what he is telling you rather than to how he is telling it.

What do I say to him when he is teased by his friends or his classmates?

"Children get teased about many things... even the way they eat a hamburger."

Teasing is a common problem that most children have to deal with as a part of growing up. If they are not teased about their speech, they likely will be teased about something else—for example, the color of their hair, the glasses they wear or even the way they eat a hamburger. Undoubtedly, your child (like all children) will experience his share of teasing. In any event, he needs to be helped to understand about teasing generally. Then, it will be easier for him to figure out how to handle it.

You can help by listening and talking to him about his feelings about being teased. Also, you can discuss together the things one can do when teased. You can even talk about the way you felt and the things you did when you were teased as a child. Another thing you can do is to help him focus his attention on other things. For example, go for an ice cream cone, suggest he call a close friend, discuss plans for an upcoming event, and so forth.

As I talk to children about the teasing they do, they explain to me that they are not trying to be mean or to hurt one's feelings. They are just "kidding around." They say that they only "kid around" with their friends. They don't kid around with those they don't like or don't know. In my experience, most "teasing" is of this kind. You can work with your child to help him to decide the best way to handle it. If there is one child or a small group who tease to be cruel, then often it is best to discuss with the teacher, and, if necessary, the school counselor the best ways to handle it.

What do I say to his teachers?

"No one interrupts, talks for or finishes words for anyone else."

It is a good idea to make an appointment to meet your child's classroom teacher before classes begin. Teachers welcome the chance to discuss stuttering openly with parents. It will help the teacher to decide the most reasonable ways to handle your child's speech in the classroom if she learns how you have been handling it at home. She can appreciate the fact that you have talked to your child about hesitations, repetitions and other disruptions in speech as "mistakes we make while learning to talk." Also, that the related physical tensing and struggling (if present) are efforts to fight or hide the mistakes. After all, the teacher's job is to help children learn. Teachers know how upset some children become when they don't do things "right."

The teacher will want to know that at home you encourage your child to say what he wants to say even though he has some disruptions while saying it. You will want to tell the teacher that you listen to what he says, not react to how he says it. You compliment him—not for speaking fluently, but for an interesting observation of good talking manners in the home. No one interrupts, talks for, or finishes words for anyone else.

You will want to learn from the teacher the kinds of oral recitation (oral reading, short answers, oral reports) the children perform. It will be helpful if you then talk about this with your child so he knows what to expect. Suggest to the teacher that she do the same thing. You both can learn the way he feels about it—the parts that don't worry him and the parts that do. Then you and the teacher can discuss the best ways to help him meet oral recitations constructively.

Are there classroom activities that can help children who stutter?

There are simple, common sense adjustments that teachers can make to routine classroom activities that have been found to be helpful to other children. These include:

Oral Presentations in School

(a) If the child is fearful of reciting orally, his reading assignments can be sent home. You can have him practice reading them alone to you. This enables him to gain confidence of knowing all of the words, and it gives him the experience of hearing his voice as he reads.

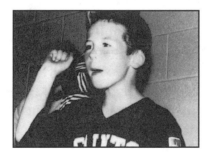

Answering Questions in School

(b) If he is afraid of being asked questions to be answered aloud, you can pretend to be the teacher and ask him to answer questions aloud. This enables him to practice taking the time to answer, to revise an answer, and generally to "think on his feet" out loud.

Telling Stories in School

(c) If he is afraid of activities involving telling a story or giving an oral report, he can prepare it and present it to you— and perhaps to other members of the family.

If the teacher knows the things you are doing at home, she can plan her activities with the child accordingly. As much as possible, the teacher should ask the child to recite just as she does any other child in the classroom.

If speech therapy is recommended, indicate to the speech clinician and to the teacher that you will cooperate in every way possible.

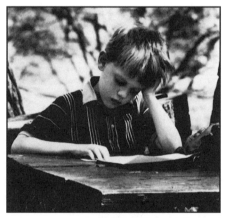

photo credit: paul diamond

Things that Teachers can do to help

General Practice

1) Meeting parents of a child who stutters before or near the beginning of classes will help you learn the parents' concerns and expectations.
2) If there is a speech clinician at your school, contact her to see what suggestions she may have for this child. If she is working with him, find out what her objectives are.
3) Don't let the child who stutters get away with things just because he stutters.
4) As much as possible, treat the child who stutters the same as the other children in your class—with the exception of special assistance with oral recitation, for example, allowing him a bit more time to do his recitation and focus on the message of his recitation not **how** he delivers the message!
5) Children who stutter should be expected to perform all classroom oral recitations even though they may need some special help to succeed.
6) Talk with the child about the class's oral recitation requirements, how she feels about it and what you can do to help.
7) Encourage the child to practice his oral recitation requirements at home.

Communication

1) Allow children who stutter enough time to talk; they may

    frequently have trouble starting to talk.
2) Encourage good talking manners in the classroom, no one interrupts, talks for or finishes words for anyone else.
3) Make it clear to the entire class that disfluencies are part of learning to talk. Ridiculing, teasing, or mocking others when they struggle to learn does not help, and often hinders the person. As much as possible, make the classroom a no-ridicule zone!

Keep in Mind

Know that your caring enough to do these things can make a big difference!

Chapter 5

what is involved in therapy?

Hugo H. Gregory, Ph.D.

Therapy can take many forms. It may consist of a few sessions with parents, or it may involve a longer relationship of working with both the parents and the child for several months. In general, the older the child, the longer therapy will take. With a preschool child, the clinician tries to prevent or minimize stuttering. The older the child when therapy begins, the less likely all traces of the problem can be eliminated, at least quickly. This chapter provides information about what is involved in therapy and deals with questions you may have about how therapy can help.

How are decisions made about what is needed?

In general, deciding from what a child needs in therapy involves: (1) the ways in which your child's speech differs that of most children, and (2) what circumstances in his speech development or environment are contributing to the problem.

"Some children who stutter may also have other speech problems."

Specifically, we are more concerned about a child who has more (1) one syllable word repetitions ("I,I,I" "He,He,He") and/or

(2) breaks within words (sound repetitions "M,M,M,Mama," syllable repetitions "Mama,ma,mama," sound prolongations "MMMMama"). Noticeable physical tension (that may be seen or heard) in the lips, jaw, larynx or chest areas accompanying these repetitions and prolongations, or blocks in the child's speech, are more certain signs of a stuttering problem.

If stuttering has been present for more than six months, and if it seems to be coming more constant from day to day, and more consistent from one situation to the next, more than just parent guidance is likely to be recommended.

If stress in the way the parents and others talk to the child or stress in the way family members relate to each other is contributing to increased stuttering, then these stresses must be reduced.

Circumstances That May Increase Stuttering	
Communicative Stress	Interpersonal Stress
The Way Parents and Others Talk with the Child	The Way Familiy Members Relate to Each Other
1. Rapid speech rates and fast-paced conversation 2. Interrupting the child 3. Guessing what the child is about to say and then saying it for him 4. Beginning to speak immediately when the child pauses or stops talking 5. Bombarding the child with many questions 6. Competing to get into an ongoing conversation	1. Unrealistic demands on the child 2. Conflict about discipline 3. Hectic or inconsistent family routine 4. Fast-paced family life 5. Experiences that make the child feel "put down" 6. Consistent as well as strong disapproval for any and all mistakes

What if the child has other speech and language problems?

Some children who stutter may also have other speech problems. They may have trouble pronouncing some sounds or words, or they may have trouble choosing words quickly and correctly. Some may have trouble quickly and correctly using grammar. Since these other speech problems could be related to the development of stuttering or could complicate treatment, therapy may need to focus on these problems when it is appropriate.

At what age should a child be evaluated or receive therapy?

Ordinarily, parents don't get concerned about a child's speech—"Is my child beginning to stutter? "—until at least 24 to 36 months of age when the child uses sufficient language to speak in sentences. Whenever parents are concerned about a child's speech, it is time to see a speech clinician who works with children. If it is a question about stuttering, parents should seek a speech clinician who includes stuttering as one of the areas in which he/she is specialized (ideally a speech clinician who has received Board-certified Specialty Recognition in Fluency Disorders).

"Talking seems a little harder for you today."

How can I tell if my child knows he is stuttering?

A child just beginning to stutter may say "Why can't I talk?" or "I can't say it." We cannot be sure just what this means in terms of awareness. But if he talks about it several times a week, he is probably becoming more aware. If the child stops talking when he is having trouble or changes his speech in some ways, for example by whispering, this is a more certain sign that he is aware that he is stuttering.

There is nothing wrong with occasionally commenting about obvious speech difficulty by saying, "All people have trouble talking sometimes. You are still learning how to talk." Or you may say, "Talking seems a little harder for you today." **It is important to acknowledge the difficulty the child is experiencing.**

How are parents involved in therapy?

Since the home environment has a very strong influence on the child's speech, it is clear that the parents are going to be involved in therapy.

Early in the process, we find that parents have many questions about speech development and stuttering. We describe the development of speech from words to phrases to sentences, and help them to identify the ways in which the smooth flow of speech may be disrupted (sound repetitions or prolongations, syllable repetitions, blocks, etc.)

"I like the way you are taking turns."

As the parents describe those situations that seem to increase or decrease their child's stuttering, we instruct them how to chart episodes of increased stuttering.

The following chart illustrates this procedure in the common situation where mother and father are talking and the child interrupts them:

Situation	What Did the Child Do?	Child's Speech	Child's Awareness	Cause of Child's Speech Disruption	What Did Parents Do?
Mother and Father are talking	Interrupted. Wanted Father's attention	Repeated syllables prolonged sounds in tense way	Excited, but unaware of speech problems	The child wants immediate attention. Can't wait.	Father said "I'll listen as soon as your mother and I are through talking." And he did.
Start →	(Parent-child communicative behaviors during conversation)				→ End

41

How are parents helped to better manage speaking situations in the home?

In the illustration above, we worked with parents for better ways to manage the situation. Here, the speech clinician suggested having "talking times" with the

"The clinician arranges for changes to be made in small steps..."

child. Then the parents were advised to have times at home in which mother and father listened carefully to the child and emphasized each having a turn to talk. When the child did this too, he was encouraged by being told, "I like the way you are taking turns." As progress was made, taking turns was discussed with other family members. The goal was to give the child more attention in a structured way and to help him learn how to take part in a conversation without interrupting others.

We as speech clinicians not only tell but also show the parents what changes to make. We may demonstrate a more relaxed, slightly slower rate of speaking, pausing longer after the child speaks before responding. Gradually, parents take over more of the clinician's role and use the changed behavior when talking with the child. Children respond better when they know that their parents are learning too.

Isn't it hard for parents to change their behavior?

Yes it is, and it is also very important. This is why the clinician arranges for changes to be made in small steps and provides opportunities for practice at the clinic before any attempt is made to make changes at home. In a group session, parents often share with other parents some of their questions, frustrations, and successes. Most parents want to learn to respond appropriately, and once they get into the process of change, it is rewarding. The best reward for the parents is to see their child's speech improving and to feel they can do something to help.

How does the clinician work with the child?

Pre-school-age children

When a child is seen in the very early stages of beginning to stutter, parental guidance or counseling will usually be the approach used. Some clinicians want to always take a look at changing the child's environment before working more directly with the child. Some suggest permissive, warm, sharing, comfortable speaking situations in the clinic along with parental guidance. Additional observations of the child can be made in this atmosphere which is usually conducive to more relaxed speech.

The clinician makes a decision about more direct therapy with the child taking into consideration:

1) the amount of tension in the child's speech,

2) how long the problem has existed,

3) how constant the child's speaking difficulties are, and

4) whether or not there are other related problems of speech.

For example, if the problem has been present for less than a year, stuttering is still what we call a borderline problem, and there are no complicating speech problems, then the child may be seen on a short term basis (4 to 10 sessions), The parents can watch the clinician working with the child and can do such things as those listed below:

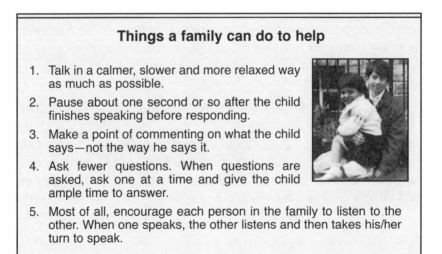

Things a family can do to help

1. Talk in a calmer, slower and more relaxed way as much as possible.

2. Pause about one second or so after the child finishes speaking before responding.

3. Make a point of commenting on what the child says—not the way he says it.

4. Ask fewer questions. When questions are asked, ask one at a time and give the child ample time to answer.

5. Most of all, encourage each person in the family to listen to the other. When one speaks, the other listens and then takes his/her turn to speak.

Recently, when a father saw me doing this with his child, he said, "I know I have always been energetic and excited when playing with Tony. I thought that was the way to get his interest. I just never thought about how that could be related to his stuttering."

When the pattern of stuttering is more firmly established, even in preschool children, the clinician may help these children change their speech by showing them (modeling) an easier, more relaxed manner of speaking beginning with shorter and working up to longer sentences/phrases.

An important point to remember: To get the most out of therapy, parents must learn to model for the child, just like the clinician does!

School-Age Children

"I can tell my speech what to do."

With older school children, the clinician can more directly show the child how to reduce tension and speak in a more easy relaxed way with smooth movements between words. Of course, therapy is different with each child. Sometimes, just showing the child—beginning with words and working up to longer phrases—how to speak in a slower, more relaxed manner is enough. With others, we may contrast "easy talking" with "hard talking," and in those where there is more tension (and the child expects more difficulty) on certain sounds or words, we help the child to be more aware of tension and contrast this with the easier more relaxed way. As one eight-year-old youngster said to me, "I can tell my speech what to do."

The school-age child's attitudes are dealt with in two ways: (1) by explaining to them how speech is produced and by helping them to see that changing speech is like learning a skill in a sport (hitting a ball) and, (2) by being a good listener and helping the child better understand and deal with his worries and concerns, such as teasing by a peer.

What about the parents' role in therapy at school?

School speech clinicians often say that it is difficult to do successful therapy in the schools because they cannot counsel parents as needed. Children are so much more successful when they have their parents' support and realize that their mother and father know what they are doing in therapy. Parents can learn to reinforce what their child is learning as they themselves learn what to do to help their child! The school speech clinician, the teachers, and the parents should be a team in working with the school-age child who stutters.

How much therapy is needed?

This depends on the many factors described above. When a decision has been made to see both parents and child for therapy, it is best for therapy to be fairly intensive at first, that is at least three individual sessions of 30-50 minutes a week. In most cases, the frequency of therapy is typically reduced as the child improves. However, sometimes intensive treatment is not possible, with once-a-week treatment being effective, although perhaps taking longer to achieve the same result.

How long will it take?

It may only take a few weeks with a preschool child just beginning to stutter. With a more developed problem in either a preschool or school age child, therapy may take between 9 to 24 months, sometimes more. Since so many circumstances affect speech, it is important that children be followed carefully for several years following therapy. During this time, the parents and the clinician should stay in touch. In this way, "therapy" for a child who stutters could last well beyond the time when the child/parents are coming for weekly therapy sessions.

When is consultation with another professional, such as a psychologist, needed?

In discussing the environment of the child, we have referred to interpersonal stress related to increased stuttering. Some examples of these stress factors are:

1) Parents who have unrealistic levels of expectation for their children's behavior such as neatness and table manners (these parents often have high levels of expectation for speech development).

2) Sibling rivalries or discipline practices that are causing conflict.

3) Hectic or inconsistent family routines.

4) Parents who are anxious about child rearing practices or have feelings of guilt about how they have reacted to their child's speech.

"Circumstances surrounding a stuttering problem in a child are often fairly complex..."

5) Some basic unhappiness in a marriage.

When the speech clinician sees that stress factors such as these are consistently interfering with progress in therapy, a referral to a psychologist (preferably one interested in children with speech problems) for evaluation may provide helpful insight. Such referrals may indicate that another treatment like family therapy or psychotherapy for the child or parents is needed.

Oftentimes parents do not accept this advice. Some clinics employ a multidisciplinary approach in which the child who stutters and parents are always seen by a psychologist. Circumstances surrounding a stuttering problem in a child are often fairly complex, and input from other professionals is often very helpful to the child, family and speech clinician.

How much success can be expected?

Success rates are very high when therapy begins during the period of two to five years of age. They are even better when parents have taken proper steps when they were first concerned. With school age children, it is less likely that fluency can be completely normalized. If the child reacts with frustration to the therapy process, it may be best to postpone treatment until later. If the child does not appear to be benefiting from therapy, the speech clinician should be able to explain why, and you should have the kind of relationship with the clinician in which the reasons can be discussed freely. Consultation with another clinician should be considered.

Who should we go to for therapy?

You should seek a speech clinician who includes stuttering as one of the areas in which he/she is specialized. Ideally, you will want to find a speech clinician with board-certified recognition as having specialty/expertise in stuttering. More and more clinicians are specializing in stuttering.

Talk to more than one professional before you choose. When you have narrowed your choices, consult with some of the clinicians' colleagues about their reputations. This is an important decision. It involves your time and your money, and most of all your child's future.

How much will therapy cost?

Private practitioners charge from seventy-five to one hundred and fifty dollars per hour. Most often the fee will be eighty to one hundred dollars an hour. Total cost could be from one to several thousand dollars. Of course, in the case of short-term treatment such as that described for some children beginning to stutter, it could be less.

University clinics where students are being trained or publicly supported institutions charge on a sliding scale according to ability to pay, and the therapy will be less expensive. For example, the range might be from twenty to eighty dollars an hour.

You should be satisfied with progress as therapy proceeds and feel free to inquire about the prognosis and costs. Health insurance policy coverage of stuttering therapy varies. You should consult with your insurance agent and request that the speech clinician send reports or any other required information to the company.

For more information on how to deal with insurance claims, call the Stuttering Foundation toll free number, 800-992-9392, or see page 60.

Chapter 6

what if my child continues to stutter?

Barry Guitar, Ph.D.

If your child's stuttering persists after treatment, you may have questions about how it will affect him. You may wonder how it will influence his social development and his school achievement as well as his future happiness. You may also want to know what you can do that will help. Our answers to these questions, given in this section, are based on experiences with many children with a wide variety of stuttering problems. The vast majority of these children have continued to improve their speech as they grew older with the help and support of their parents.

"Many brilliant scientists and writers...were people who stutter."

What should I do if he still stutters after therapy?

Speech-language therapy with young children can result in stuttering's being cured or reduced so much that it is hardly noticeable. If your child has had therapy and has improved, he may still slip from time to time, however. For example, your child may stutter a little when he is excited or tired. He may also stutter some when telling a long, complex story. He may also stutter when describing some event that took place outside of or elsewhere in the house. Be accepting of some slippage. Even if he slips a lot, show him you really care about him regardless of whether he stutters or not. When he talks with you, try to listen attentively to his message, try to focus on **what** he is saying not **how** he is saying it.

If your child is stuttering mildly, and for brief periods, it isn't likely to bother him. He will probably be able to handle it, especially if you are supportive. On the other hand, if your child is stuttering enough so that he is tensing pretty hard to get words out, or avoids talking, he may need further therapy. If you aren't sure, check with the clinician who worked with him before.

Sometimes, going back for a booster session of therapy will be enough to get him back on track. Other times, going to a different therapist may be appropriate. See how your child feels about it.

Will continued stuttering hinder his academic success?

Many brilliant scientists and writers—for example, Charles Darwin and Lewis Carroll—were people who stuttered. Thus there is no reason to suppose that stuttering is caused by low intelligence or is associated with poor achievement. In fact, a great many people who stutter take pride in how well they did in school and college. Your child's success in school will be influenced by many individual factors, independent of stuttering, such as parental support, how bright he is as well as how motivated he is. His academic success will probably be greater if he doesn't let his stuttering keep him from participating in class.

Teachers can make a difference in this regard, too. They can encourage your child to talk despite his stuttering, and they can help him realize that they and others appreciate his ideas. It is important, therefore, that you and the school clinician stay in contact with your child's teachers to help them foster his school progress. Through this contact, you and the clinician can also inform teachers who may not understand

"Making friends is done by being friendly."

stuttering or know how to react appropriately to it. (In Chapter 3, pp. 20-21, we have discussed the many things that parents can do to help.)

If your child chooses to go to college, his stuttering should not keep him from doing so. College admissions officers are likely to welcome a student who has experienced a problem like stuttering but hasn't let it hold him back. Many colleges and universities, in fact, provide speech therapy services because they expect that some of their students will stutter or have other speech-language disorders.

Will stuttering keep him from making friends?

No. Making friends is done by being friendly. Your child may find it a little harder to talk to other kids his age, but as long as he listens to and talks with other children in a friendly way, he will make and have friends.

Many of the children who stutter that I know have plenty of friends because they are a lot of fun. They like other people and they have a good sense of humor. They don't let their stuttering keep them from being talkative and playful.

I have worked with kids who stuttered only a little but were at first so worried about their stuttering that they didn't talk a lot. Their parents worried too, and that didn't help. As we worked together, these kids loosened up. They learned to be less bothered when they were teased about their stuttering. They talked about their stuttering to other kids. They also began to get interested in other kids which naturally led to making friends.

Will my child be able to play sports?

Absolutely. Some of the most talented athletes of this decade are people who stutter. For example, Bob Love, Lester Hayes, Bo Jackson, Ken Venturi, Bill Walton and Ron Harper are all stutterers as well as superstars. Of course very few of us are going to be that talented athletically. But if your child likes to play sports, he'll find it rewarding. If he's good, or just enthusiastic, other kids will enjoy playing sports with him. That, in turn, will boost his confidence, which may help his speech.

And non-team sports like karate, tennis, etc., if your child is interested and enjoys them, are wonderful confidence builders as well.

Children who stutter often feel most free when they are able to lose themselves in something that doesn't focus on speech, like sports or other physical activities. Stuttering often disappears or becomes very mild when a child plays sports. Even a child who severely stutters can usually yell just about anything to his teammates during the excitement of a game.

What does the future hold if his stuttering persists into adolescence and beyond?

You may be thinking far into the future, wondering about whether your child would have any problems dating, marrying, or bringing

"Dating for teenagers can be hard at first, whether they stutter or not."

up children. The answer is that he will probably have no more problems than someone who doesn't stutter. Let's take this one step at a time, first dating, then marriage and then adulthood, in general.

How will stuttering influence his or her dating?

Dating, for teenagers, can be hard at first, whether they stutter or not. Most teenagers who stutter learn to go ahead and make friends with members of the opposite sex despite their stuttering. They find out that if they are friendly, their approach is usually successful. Whether a real relationship develops is a matter of chemistry and common interests. Stuttering doesn't get in the way once two people get to know each other. Nor does it get in the way of a relationship that leads to marriage.

Will stuttering influence his or her ability to get married?

Stuttering is also no barrier to having a happy marriage and raising a family. It is true that children of people who stutter may inherit an increased vulnerability to stuttering, but most will not stutter. Even if they do, parents who stutter themselves usually know what responses are most helpful to a child who may begin to stutter. They have good ideas about how to talk about stuttering with their children. They can be objective and can share feelings about stuttering. They can create a home environment that nurtures the growth of fluent speech.

Will stuttering influence my child in other ways when he or she gets older?

You may wonder if your child's stuttering will become more of a problem as he grows older in other ways than marriage and a family. Perhaps you know someone who stutters severely and for whom stuttering is a problem. It is important for you to know that it doesn't have to be this way. For example, I stutter on many occasions, but I speak in public, meet new people easily, talk on the telephone, do all the things that normally fluent speakers do. Most of the time I speak fairly easily, but occasionally I get hung up on a stutter. My listeners usually take their cues from how I react. When I keep my cool despite stuttering, my listeners hardly notice the stuttering. Sure, some people are impatient, but I have learned not to let them get me down. Besides, these listeners are impatient with all talkers, not just people who stutter!

There are days when stuttering does get in my way. I go through periods when my stuttering flares up for reasons I don't always understand. I sometimes avoid words I might stutter on or situations that are hard for me when I know I shouldn't. Sometimes I might feel discouraged. This aspect of stuttering is a real annoyance, but it is some-

"...you always have the opportunity to let your child know he's OK as he is, whether he stutters or not."

thing I have learned to deal with. Most other adults who stutter learn to deal with it too.

What can I do that will help my child now?

If your child's stuttering persists after therapy, there are things you can do that will help him. Perhaps the most important advice we can give you is what we have said before: **accept** your child as he is regardless of the fact his stuttering has returned. Try to find out if there are new stresses or a return of old ones. Try to recall if there were things that you were doing when your child was in therapy (but are no longer doing!). Perhaps you have forgotten some of the things that were helpful—for example, speaking slowly and easily when talking to your child. Can you do those again? For more specific ideas, see the Stuttering Foundation's DVD *Stuttering and Your Child: Help for Parents* (DVD #0073). If you have seen it before, watch it again for reminders of what you can do to help your child. You can also watch helpful videos online at www.stutteringhelp.org.

Although you are probably one of the most important influences on how your child responds to his stuttering, there may be other people who affect your child's stuttering and his feelings. One example is people who are impatient with him because of his stuttering. Sometimes you can speak to them in private to help them change their behavior. Many times, however, you can't intervene in time. But you always have the opportunity to let your child know he's OK as he is, whether he stutters or not.

If he is having a particularly bad time with his stuttering, he may feel down in the dumps. You can help a lot here by encouraging him to talk about how he feels. Your child may feel frustrated or angry or hurt because of his stuttering. Being able to share these feelings can make it easier for him. Try to sense what he's feeling by his facial expression and tone of voice.

> *"Support your little messenger by listening to his message rather than how he delivers it."*

Share with him that you also have had temporary feelings of sadness or anger.

When your child's stuttering bothers you, and it surely will on some days, try to remember that some of his reactions to his stuttering are determined by those around him. If you can foster in your family an acceptance of your child's stuttering and other speech-language mistakes and problems, your child will be likely to struggle with it less and less. He will learn to talk confidently in spite of it.

If my child continues to stutter somewhat, can I really help him?

Yes, you can, As we've already said, if your child still stutters after therapy, you can help him in several ways:

First, be **accepting** of your child even if his stuttering bothers you. Show your caring—especially when his stuttering seems worst. That is when he needs you most.

Second, **encourage** your child in all ways to be himself. Your efforts will show him that stuttering is only one part of his life.

Third, when he talks with you, **support** your little messenger by listening to his message rather than how he delivers it.

Doing these things will really help!

If the child continues to stutter, things to remember:

1) Many highly successful people continue to stutter into their teen and adult years.
2) Making friends occurs by being friendly, not by being fluent!
3) Children who stutter can and do participate in all events—sports, academics, etc.—that their abilities and interests permit.
4) People who stutter are just as apt as those who do not to successfully date, marry and raise children.
5) Parents can be the biggest help by accepting their child, supporting him and letting him share his feelings with you.
6) Above all, support and listen to the message of your little messenger rather than how he delivers it!

---

Chapter 7

should we seek help?

William H. Perkins, Ph.D.

Won't therapy make him more aware of his problem? Make his problem worse?

For years, everyone (many professionals included) tiptoed around stuttering as if we were walking on eggs for fear of calling attention to the problem. Many presumed that this would make it worse. No longer. You should consider two things.

For one thing, if your child's stuttering is developing into a problem for him, he is already becoming aware of it and is frustrated by it. When parents pretend nothing is wrong, he may conclude that his stuttering is so bad they can't even talk about it.

The second consideration is that early treatment has shown the best results of all. Instead of making stuttering worse, the sooner effective help is provided after stuttering is first noticed, the better the child's chances of full recovery. If stuttering continues after puberty, it usually persists in one form or another.

Will he be cured?

If stuttering does persist into adulthood, he may hope for a cure, but hardly anyone, neither *"With children, the prospects are much better."* professionals nor people who stutter, realistically expects a great deal more than improvement. These adults may be able to sound normal much of the time, but most continue to think of themselves as people who stutter.

With children, the prospects are much better. By helping them before they begin to fear stuttering and develop reactions to it—fear and reactions which can complicate the lives of adults who stutter—these children have a good chance of becoming reasonably normal speakers. They may still stumble and hesitate in their speech from time to time, but that happens to everyone.

The important thing is that these children not feel so frustrated by their speech mistakes, hesitations and bobbles that speaking becomes a struggle, and they begin to identify themselves as stutterers. Prevention of a self-image of being a person who stutters goes a long way towards what could be called a cure for stuttering. Beginning therapy as soon as the problem becomes apparent goes a long way toward prevention.

Where do we begin to seek help?

"...most speech clinicians refer for specialized problems like stuttering."

First you need to find a specialist who has up-to-date knowledge of stuttering. Although any speech clinician licensed by the state or certified by the American Speech-Language-Hearing Association has at least minimal qualifications to provide professional help for stuttering, most refer this problem to clinicians who have specialized in it. For much the same reason even though legally qualified, most licensed physicians who have not specialized in surgery refer patients to a surgeon. Likewise, most speech clinicians refer for specialized problems like stuttering. Universities and colleges with training programs in speech pathology (communication disorders) will be able to direct you to such specialists, as will the Stuttering Foundation of America, which is devoted exclusively to serving the interests of people who stutter.

What do I ask my pediatrician? Whose advice should we take?

Pediatricians have specialized knowledge of the health problems of children, so all questions concerning your child's health should be directed to them. Stuttering, however, is not a problem about which most physicians have adequate information, but they usually know a speech clinician to whom they routinely refer a wide variety of speech and language disorders. However, you would be well advised to determine if these speech clinicians are specialized in as well as successful in treating children who stutter. If they are not, then ask them for a referral to someone who is.

What if I'm told that my child who stutters will "outgrow it?"

The chances are good that he will. Approximately eighty percent of children whose parents think they have stuttered will stop before adulthood, and most of these will before puberty.

It's the risk that your child may be one of the 20% that won't that you need to consider. First, was it a specialist in stuttering who told you he is "likely to outgrow it?" Predicting whether a child will recover or persist in stuttering is difficult. It requires expert knowledge, experience and training.

The reason you may want to begin therapy early, rather than wait, is that his chances of full recovery decrease the older he grows. If in doubt, you have much to gain and little to lose by starting treatment as early as possible.

If we are uncomfortable with the help we receive for our child, should we seek a second opinion?

Yes, by all means. You would be wise to seek a second opinion even if you're not uncomfortable with the first. And if you're still

"Even the best authorities have honest differences of opinion."

uncomfortable seek a third opinion. Diagnosis and treatment are far from being exact sciences. Even the best authorities have honest differences of opinion, so it pays you to find out what more than one expert thinks.

If therapy is recommended, can he receive it at school?

Many schools do have clinicians who work successfully with children who stutter. Compared to the frequency of occurrence of other speech and language disorders, school clinicians see stuttering relatively infrequently, so they may not have much experience treating children who stutter.

Here are two suggestions for finding out if your school clinician can provide the necessary help. The first is to ask the parents of a

"Look for signs of gradual improvement, not a quick cure."

stuttering child, who was treated by your potential clinician, what their experience was. See what did and did not seem to help them and their child. The other is to try speech-language therapy at school. Be sure, however, with therapy at school, as with all therapists, to give it sufficient time to show some influence, for example, at least 3 months or more.

How soon will we know if he's being helpful?
What should we look for?

With young children, positive changes begin to appear sometimes within weeks, certainly within several months. It is important to remember: Look for signs of gradual improvement, not a quick cure. As long as he is feeling better about himself, about his speech, and increasingly enjoys talking, you are on the right track. If he continues to struggle to speak, to avoid certain words and situations, to not want to talk at school or at home—these are signs that therapy is not helping much. Again, give therapy a fair trial, at least several months, before passing judgment.

Will he have to go every day?

Intensive therapy (three or more times a week) has advantages, so if the opportunity for frequent therapy is available, take it. This is especially true for older children at the beginning of treatment. Later sessions can be spaced farther apart without slowing progress.

Intensive therapy may not be available, however, especially at school. This certainly doesn't mean therapy won't be successful, but it does mean it will probably take longer.

"The longest journey...starts with a single step...you have taken that step by reading this book."

Above all **remember,** if a problem exists, seek professional advice and help. Early treatment for stuttering can and does help.

The longest journey, it is said, starts with a single step. You have taken that step by reading this book. Now that you've taken that step, take another one. Ask for professional assistance, if you believe your child needs it. It can really help you reach your destination of having your child become a more normally fluent speaker!

No matter how long your child receives therapy, chances are very good it will help. Together with your love and guidance, there is every reason to believe that your child can be helped to become a more fluent speaker. [For additional advice on how you can help, view the films mentioned in Chapter 6 and read If Your Child Stutters: A Guide for Parents, *Book #0011, available from the Stuttering Foundation of America, www.stutteringhelp.org.]*

Obtaining Reimbursement for Stuttering Treatment

Approximately three million children and adults in the U.S. stutter. This guide provides suggestions and resources for obtaining payment for the treatment of stuttering.

1. Will my health plan cover stuttering treatment?

Before contacting your health plan, review your policy for coverage looking for such terms as "speech therapy," "speech-language pathology," "physical therapy and other rehabilitation services," or "other medically necessary services or therapies." A phone call to the health plan can confirm your interpretation of coverage. Document the name of the person with whom you speak as well as dates and times.

Provide the health plan with information about the neurological basis of stuttering; the available evidence states that stuttering is a "disorder associated with left inferior frontal structural anomalies" (*Brain*, 2009) and that " adults with persistent stuttering ... (have) anatomical irregularities in the areas of the brain that control language and speech" (*Neurology*, July 24, 2001). Children who stutter demonstrate atypical brain anatomy as well (*Neuroimage*, February, 2008).

When speaking with the health plan representative, it may be helpful to provide the appropriate diagnostic code for the type of stuttering you are seeking treatment coverage for. There are some recent changes in the relevant diagnostic codes. While the **default code has typically been 307.0** for all forms of stuttering, **new codes are scheduled to take effect in October 2010.** These will include a **new "default" code** of **315.35** for **"Childhood onset fluency disorder"** to include most cases of stuttering and cluttering. **Adult onset** stuttering, which is relatively rare, will be covered by the codes **438.14** for **stuttering following stroke,** and **784.52** for **fluency disorder secondary to other medical conditions.** The prior default code **(307.0)** will only be used for **stuttering not described by these other codes.** The treatment codes for stuttering include **92506** for **speech evaluation,** 92507 for **individual speech treatment,** and 92508 for **group speech treatment.**

Be sure to get the name of the health plan representative with whom you talked and ask for confirmation of coverage in writing. Specifics of coverage (e.g., any limit on the number of sessions, co-payments, deductible amounts, etc.) should also be provided in writing. The health plan should provide this written notification within 30 to 60 days.

If treatment for stuttering is not covered by your policy, ask the health plan to explain the reasons for the denial in writing. This information can be helpful in appealing the original determination. Keep copies of all correspondence and detailed records of all verbal communication.

Sometimes health plans decline to cover conditions in the 315 "series" of codes, because they consider them "developmental". If you receive such a response, it is important to emphasize that the 315.35 code specifically includes the wording "childhood onset" to make it clear that "stuttering evolves before puberty, usually between two and five years of age, without apparent brain damage or other known cause" (PloS Biology, February, 2004). It impairs previously normal fluency.

2. Does the health plan require a physician referral before payment for the treatment of stuttering?

Some insurers do require this pre-approval. Your policy booklet or your insurance representative should be able to tell you if your policy requires a referral from your primary physician prior to beginning treatment for stuttering. Pre-approval may be a form that your primary physician completes and submits to the health plan. Pre-approval may also require a letter of referral, which is submitted along with your insurance form to the health plan.

If a letter is required for pre-approval of treatment for stuttering, it should contain the following information:

_____ is a patient of mine who stutters. This interferes with his/her oral communication. In order to treat this disorder, it is medically necessary that my patient receive specialized, comprehensive speech treatment from_____.

Typically, the health plan also requires a form from the speech-language pathologist, which includes the diagnostic and treatment codes for stuttering, projected treatment dates or number of treatment sessions anticipated, as well as associated fees. The health plan is required to notify you within 30 to 60 days as to the status of approval.

3. How do I submit a claim?

Speech treatment for stuttering is usually conducted in one of two ways: weekly sessions or intensive, short-term treatment programs.

A. Weekly Sessions

If speech treatment is provided once or twice a week, claims can be submitted in a number of ways: at the completion of each session, after a block of sessions, or filed with a projected number of sessions. If more sessions are needed than originally anticipated, a progress report is submitted to the health plan with a request for coverage for additional sessions. The speech-language pathologist can assist you in determining the best way to submit your claim, or may submit the claim for you.

B. Intensive Short-Term Treatment

If treatment is provided through an intensive short-term treatment program, the claim must be submitted at the completion of the program. Intensive shortterm treatment programs are typically conducted over a 2-4 week period.

Once the treatment program is completed, the speech-language pathologist will supply the appropriate diagnostic and treatment codes and either you or the clinician will submit this information, along with your insurance form, to the health plan.

Regardless of the type of treatment program recommended-weekly or intensive, short-term-you should call the health plan a week after mailing the claim to make certain it has been received.

4. What can I do if my claim is denied?

If your claim is denied, request the reasons for denial in writing. You have the right to appeal the denial. Remember, persistence often pays off.

First, write a letter stating your intention to appeal the denial. The health plan may request additional information about the treatment and/or they may ask for an objective measurement of progress. They may cite as a reason for denial that treatment is "educational in nature" or that treatment is not "medically necessary." Your appeal must address the specific reasons for denial.

An appeal letter typically includes a description of the disorder and its medical nature. A copy of the physician's referral letter (if pre-approval was needed) should be included. It may be helpful to quote those sections of the policy booklet that describe the coverage for speech-language pathology treatment, if it helps your case. Then you will need to describe how the treatment meets the policy criteria.

In any correspondence with the health plan:

- Use terms that are **medically oriented** (e.g., evaluation, diagnosis, condition) rather than behavioral or learning theory terminology (e.g., test, examination, teach).
- Do not include the time of onset of stuttering, unless specifically requested.
- Include estimated length of treatment if known.
- Indicate that treatment is provided by an ASHA-certified, and licensed (where Applicable) speech-language pathologist and include the clinician's ASHA certification number and state license number.
- Demonstrate significant practical improvement using objective, measurable terms.
- Document improvement by indicating how the patient has applied progress in treatment to real life situations (may be referred to as functional outcomes).

Your speech-language pathologist can help you with this appeal. Sample appeal letters are also available through the American Speech-Hearing-Language Association (ASHA).

Once the health plan receives the information, they must respond within a time period of 30 to 60 days depending upon the state. **Follow up and persistence can lead to success!**

5. What action can I take if my appeal is denied?

If you feel that your appeal has been unfairly denied or that your case was handled unprofessionally or inappropriately, there is action that can be taken.

- Contact your state insurance commissioner to determine if there are any other instances in which claims have been unfairly denied and/or file a complaint. Contact information for your insurance commissioner can be found by contacting the Publications Department of the National Association of Insurance Commissioners by phone (816-783-8300), by fax (816-460-7593), or online (*www.naic.org*).
- Contact the American Speech-Language-Hearing Association by phone (800-498-2071) or by e-mail (*www.asha.org*) or your state speech-language-hearing association. Your speech-language pathologist can provide you with contact information for your state speech-language-hearing association.
- Contact the Stuttering Foundation of America by phone (800-992-9392) or by e-mail (*info@stutteringhelp.org* or visit *www.stutteringhelp.org*).
- Recommend to your employer or union that coverage for speech-language treatment should be included in your health benefits plan.
- Consider filing a claim in small claims court or state court if all other efforts fail.

6. Are there any other ways to pay for treatment?

There are other ways to pay for treatment if you are having difficulty financing yourself. Here are some alternatives:

- Most states have an agency that helps handicapped or disabled individuals. The names vary from state to state but are usually called Departments of Vocational Rehabilitation. You can find your state's department by calling information at your sate capitol. Contact the agency to see if you qualify. Most states require a minimum age of 18 for vocational rehabilitation services.
- You can request financial help from your local civic organizations like the Elks Club, Lions, Rotary, SERTOMA, Etc.

Reference this material as follows: American Speech-Language-Hearing Association Special Interest Division 4, Fluency and Fluency Disorders and Stuttering Foundation of America (1998; Revised 2002, 2010). Obtaining reimbursement for stuttering treatment. Rockville MD: Author.

Risk Factors

Some factors place a child at risk for stuttering. Knowing these factors will help you try to decide whether or not your child needs to see a speech-language pathologist[1,2].

1. Family History

There is now strong evidence that almost half of all children who stutter have a family member who stutters. The risk that your child is actually stuttering instead of just having normal disfluencies increases if that family member is still stuttering. There is less risk if the family member outgrew stuttering as a child.

2. Age at onset

Children who begin stuttering before age 3½ are more likely to outgrow stuttering; if your child begins stuttering before age 3, there is a much better chance she will outgrow it within 6 months.

3. Time since onset

Between 75% and 80% of all children who begin stuttering will stop within 12 to 24 months without speech therapy. If your child has been stuttering longer than 6 months, he may be less likely to outgrow it on his own. If he has been stuttering longer than 12 months, there is an even smaller likelihood he will outgrow it on his own.

---

[1]Longitudinal research studies by Drs. Ehud Yairi and Nicoline G. Ambrose and colleagues at the University of Illinois provide excellent new information about the development of stuttering in early childhood. Their findings are helping speech-language pathologists determine who is most likely to outgrow stuttering versus who is most likely to develop a lifelong stuttering problem. Research reports include:

Yairi, E. & Ambrose, N. (1992). A longitudinal study of stuttering in children: A preliminary report. *Journal of Speech, Language, and Hearing Research, 35,* 755-760.

Ambrose, N. & Yairi, E. (1999). Normative disfluency data for early childhood stuttering. *Journal of Speech, Language, and Hearing Research, 42,* 895-909.

Yairi, E. & Ambrose, N. (1999). Early childhood stuttering I: Persistence and recovery rates. *Journal of Speech, Language, and Hearing Research, 42,* 1097-1112.

[2]Yairi, E. & Ambrose, N. (2005). *Early Childhood Stuttering: For Clinicians by Clinicians,* ProEd, Austin, TX.

4. Gender

Girls are more likely than boys to outgrow stuttering. In fact, three to four boys continue to stutter for every girl who stutters.

Why this difference? First, it appears that during early childhood, there are innate differences between boys' and girls' speech and language abilities. Second, during this same period, parents, family members, and others often react to boys somewhat differently than girls. Therefore, it may be that more boys stutter than girls because of basic differences in boys' speech and language abilities *and* differences in their interactions with others.

That being said, many boys who begin stuttering will outgrow the problem. What is important for you to remember is that if your child is stuttering right now, it doesn't necessarily mean he or she will stutter the rest of his or her life.

5. Other speech and language factors

A child who speaks clearly with few, if any, speech errors would be more likely to outgrow stuttering than a child whose speech errors make him difficult to understand. If your child makes frequent speech errors such as substituting one sound for another or leaving sounds out of words, or has trouble following directions, you should be more concerned.

The most recent findings dispel previous reports that children who begin stuttering have, as a group, lower language skills. On the contrary, there are indications that they are well within the norms or above. Advanced language skills appear to be even more of a risk factor for children whose stuttering persists.[1]

---

[1]Yairi, E. & Ambrose, N. (2005). *Early Childhood Stuttering: For Clinicians by Clinicians,* Chapter 7, Pro-Ed, Austin, TX.

Risk Factor Chart

Place a check next to each that is true for your child

Risk Factor	More likely in beginning stuttering	True for My Child
Family history of stuttering	A parent, sibling, or other family member who still stutters	
Age at onset	After age 3½	
Time since onset	Stuttering 6–12 months or longer	
Gender	Male	
Other speech-language delays	Speech sound errors, trouble being understood, or difficulty following directions	

These risk factors place children at higher risk for developing stuttering. If your child has any of these risk factors and is showing some or all of the warning signs mentioned previously, you should be more concerned. You may want to schedule a speech screening with a speech therapist who specializes in stuttering. The therapist will decide whether your child is stuttering, and then determine whether to wait a bit longer or begin treatment right away.

With your love and guidance, there is every reason to believe that your child can be helped to be a more fluent speaker.